I0412826

Disclaimer – The information in this book is for educational purposes only. Those wishing or planning to partake in any of the activities described in this book should consult their doctor and/or any other certified health professional they work with, before doing so. The author of this book assumes no liability for any adverse outcomes. This is purely an educational book

FREE Bonus Gift!

As my way of saying thank you for reading this book,
and to help you get results even quicker,

Here's a bonus audio interview I recently did
where I talk about the 7 hidden reasons
why most people _CAN'T lose weight!_

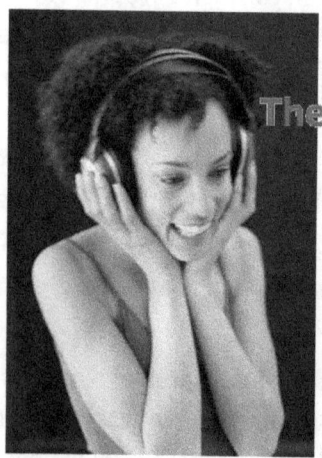

The 7 'Fat Loss Fails'

Listen to This Exclusive Interview Where I
Break Down the 7 Most Common Mistakes
You May Be Making in Your Efforts
to Lose Weight...

7 Fat Loss Fails

It's yours free!

If you've been trying to lose weight,
If you've been eating healthy, taking supplements, and
exercising regularly,
and you're _STILL_ not at your ideal weight....

**This could be _THE MOST_ valuable
thing you've ever heard!**

What You Can Expect From This Book

Real quick, before I go any further let me be very upfront with you and tell you that **losing 20lbs in 28 days *is* achievable**, but I'm not promising you that those are the results you should expect.

Why? Because, If you've grabbed this book looking for a magic pill solution, that's not what you're going to find here.

Achieving this sort of goal requires some effort. I'm not saying it's hard, I know many people who can tell you that it's actually pretty simple, but <u>it requires you to be committed to getting the results, and to follow the instructions laid-out here</u>.

In order for this to work, you'll need to be serious about making change, and you'll need to be willing to unlearn what [you think] you know about how weight loss works.

So if you're ready to learn some cool new body science and powerful strategies, and then put them to use, then this is the perfect book for you.

How to Use This Book

I've broken the book down into 3 sections to take you through the process of losing the weight.

In the 1st section I teach you the important stuff (the fundamentals) you need to know about weight loss.

This section is a very important part of your weight loss program, as it unravels a lot of road-blocks that most people run into.

In the 2nd section we'll lay out your specific weight loss program. Everything will be mapped-out and simplified, so that you know *EXACTLY* what to do moving forward.

And in the 3rd section I give you all the tactics, strategies and secrets you can put to use - right away - to start losing 20lbs in 28 days.

If you just skip to the 3 section where I teach you all of the weight-loss secrets (which is very tempting to do), you'll lack the fundamentals and a specific action plan, and any success you might have will be short-lived.

So it's very important that you read all the way through the 3 sections, so that by the end, you'll not only understand the secrets of weight loss, but also understand the fundamentals, and have a full-blown action plan.

Alright, enough talk! Let's jump in.

Section 1:

The Truth About Losing Weight

Let me start here.

You've got weight loss confused with something else entirely: Health.

The cold, hard truth about weight-loss is that it isn't understood by most people trying to lose weight - and possibly *WORSE*, it isn't understood by most "professionals" out there.

Today people are confusing weight-loss (which is a process) with a dynamic, ever-evolving, constantly-changing target we've come to label as "health".

Health VS Weight Loss

The reason I wrote this book is because people are always asking me how to lose weight. And quite often when I ask them how they're currently eating, they respond back "Oh, I eat pretty healthy!"

If you think you're going to lose weight by eating healthy – you're way off!

Don't get me wrong, we all have that one friend who just seems to be an ideal weight, but doesn't put a lot of thought or strategy into how they eat.

The problem with that is that it's not replicate'able. The same thing that worked for them, won't work for you. (You've probably tried)

It's extremely important that you understand something: Eating healthy is a philosophy, not something you can achieve.

Let me stress this...

You've got to understand this before moving to the third section of this book.

My philosophy on being healthy is different from yours, and your parents', and your best friend's, and your trainer's, and your doctor's....

Frankly....<u>Health</u> is a subject as sensitive as politics or religion.

Again, it's a philosophy - not a strategy.

However, weight loss, or more accurately fat loss, is something you do to reach a specific goal: weighing a specific amount, reaching a certain body fat percentage, or looking the way you want to look in front of the mirror.

Losing weight is a very objective, practical, *PREDICTABLE*, goal. This can be accomplished by using a strategy.

Which is more important: Nutrition or Fitness?

There are two different types of Health that people think about when they're trying to lose weight: Nutrition & Fitness

These are both categories of health that have <u>NOTHING</u> to do with weight loss.

I know that's shocking to hear, but the sooner you grasp this, the sooner you'll achieve the weight-loss results you've been looking for.

First I'm going to show you how focusing on nutrition - or eating healthy - not only prevents weight-loss, but can often lead to weight *gain*.

I see people all the time trying to achieve the practical goal of weight loss by using a philosophy about eating healthy.

Philosophy eating VS strategic eating

Think about this...

Whether you realize it or not, you've already got strong beliefs about eating. We all do, it has become part of the American culture for all of us to form beliefs about our eating & nutrition.

And depending on what your beliefs about eating are, they could be hindering your weight loss results.

I'm going to use a plain egg to illustrate how weight loss is completely different than health:

Baby Boomers VS Fitness Models

If you're over the age of 60, you probably believe that eating whole eggs is bad for your cholesterol. But if you're a bodybuilder or a fitness model, you probably believe that eggs are one of nature's most valuable, super-foods - and probably have 10 - 12 eggs per day.

Vegans VS Vegetarians

If you're a vegan, you might think of eating eggs as out-of-the-question, disgusting, or even inhumane. But if you're a common vegetarian (lacto-ovo vegetarian), eggs might be one of the only sources of complete protein you can eat to get vital nutrients into your body - making them a critical part of your diet.

Organic VS Gluten-Free

If you're an organic type of person, you might be ok with eggs, but only if there's a sticker letting you know that the government regulated how they were managed. And if you are a gluten-free type of person, you probably eat all sorts of recipes containing eggs but are more concerned with the other ingredients used with them.

Leaky Gut VS Atkins

If you're a 'Leaky Gut' type of person, you think eggs cause all sorts of health problems. But if you're an Atkins person, they're a staple part of your diet.

Grass-Fed VS Hot Dogs & Twinkies

And if you're a grass-fed type of person, you'll eat eggs, but it depends on how the mother of that egg used to eat. Or if you're a hot dog and twinkie type of person, like an ol' high-school buddy of mine, you might not even know what an egg is.

As you can see, something as simple as an egg get's very complicated when we start talking about health.

So for now - for the sake of losing weight - I need you to commit to something for me...

I need you to stop confusing weight loss with someone's philosophy about living a healthy lifestyle. Understand what a philosophy is, and what a specific strategy is, and for the time being - forget about philosophy, ok?

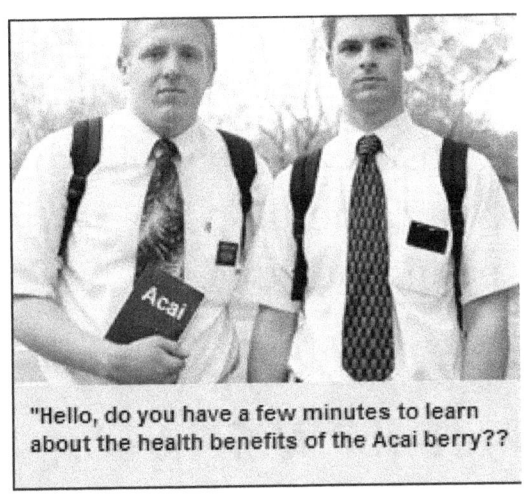

"Hello, do you have a few minutes to learn about the health benefits of the Acai berry??

Simply, learn the rules of weight loss (we'll discuss those in detail in just a minute), and then we'll use them to build your strategy.

But in case you still need a little more convincing, let me share this with you...

Why Trying to Eat Healthy Makes You Gain Weight!

The problem with philosophy-based eating is that it can be more harmful than good for you - if you're trying to lose weight.

Get this...

Here is the most common problem I see today, when it comes to people trying to lose weight by eating 'healthy'.

Gluten-Free for Weight Loss?

Let's say a friend of yours heard from Dr. Oz or Elizabeth Hasselback (the originator of the G-free craze), that gluten is bad, so they decide to begin eating gluten-free. The very first thing they do is head to the grocery store and begin searching for G-free foods.

But do they grab broccoli, or kale? Do they grab chicken or eggs?

Nope.

What they find are bars, cereals, cookies, crackers, bread, and frozen dinners that have a label telling you they are gluten-free.

The problem is, these bars, cereals, cookies, crackers, bread, and frozen dinners are all jam-packed with SUGAR! The #1 no-no for someone trying to lose weight.

Am I saying your friend shouldn't eat gluten-free? Of course not. (If they have Celiac disease then eating gluten-free is a medical necessity!)

My point here is: To eat, or not to eat gluten, is a belief system about health. It doesn't have anything to do with losing weight, and in fact - as you saw in this example - it can actually cause you to *GAIN* weight!

But don't miss the message - it's not the avoiding of gluten that leads to the weight gain. It's the focus on eating "healthy" that causes the person to overlook the #1 rule of weight loss.

Again, health and weight-loss are two totally different things. Don't confuse them.

So, if I had to give someone only one piece of advice that would help them stay focused on weight loss instead of eating "healthy", it would be this....

Avoid any foods that preach nutrients and promote health.

What does that mean?

Promoting health: Think of any foods where the label, box, or wrapper says things like "heart healthy," "recommended by doctors," "Weight Watchers approved".

Preaching Nutrients: This means any foods that say things such as: "high fiber, gluten-free, rich in antioxidants, contains vitamins, low-carb, low-sugar, low-fat".

Here's the important thing you need to remember...

Foods that are good for weight-loss (*truly* healthy foods) do NOT promote that they have health benefits. Broccoli, for example, doesn't need to convince you that it's good for you!

It's the unhealthy food companies that spend billions of advertising dollars on their labeling that try to convince you to eat them.

Do you know why people over the age of 60 think whole eggs are bad for your cholesterol?...

It was John Harvey Kellogg (co-founder of Kellogg's Corn Flakes), who lead the advertising campaign that suggested proteins (foods such as eggs) are bad for you.

His goal was to get people to stop buying eggs, and start buying corn flakes - which he promoted as the healthier alternative.

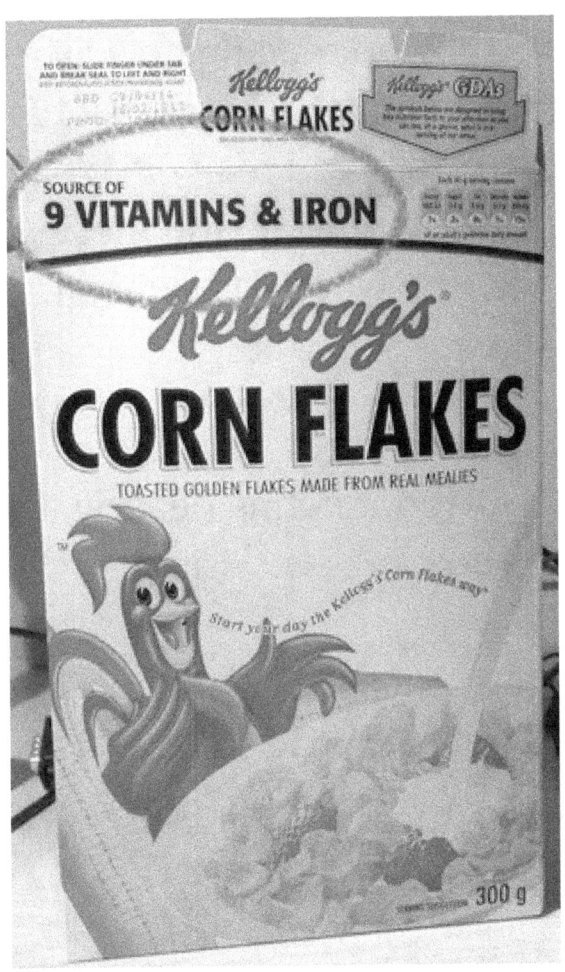

If you don't learn to spot these philosophies about eating healthy, then weight loss will always remain a mystery to you.

You'll have to keep reading new articles, and waiting to hear which foods the latest TV "health guru" tells you to avoid. You'll stay frustrated and confused, and most importantly, you won't lose weight.

But if you learn to spot - and avoid - philosophies about eating healthy, then weight loss becomes very simple.

Now let's talk about the other health philosophy: Fitness

Fitness is a Distraction

Let me be really upfront with you - I'm an advocate of fitness. I was a personal trainer for years, and loved it!

I like being fit, I think it's important, and I believe it's something that everyone should strive for. But....

Fitness is <u>NOT</u> Weight Loss

These two subjects are so often mixed, intertwined and confused – it amazes me.

Fitness is about how you feel, how your body functions, how much strength, endurance, and flexibility you have. It's about vitality, getting sick less often, healing more quickly.

You **can** have all of that and be lean (i.e. lose weight), but you can also have all of that and *NOT* be lean.

The process of becoming fit is completely different than the process of losing weight.

Let me give you an example I see all the time...

Marathon runners have belly fat

Back before I understood weight loss, there was a point in my life (my early 20's) where I was a big-time runner.

I had gotten it into my head that if I ran enough (and if I did enough crunches) I would get six pack abs. So, I began training for a marathon, and was doing two 20-minute sessions of ab exercises every-single-day.

But I noticed something happening that really baffled and irritated me:

I had more belly fat than ever!

This led me to begin studying the difference between fitness and weight loss. And I found out the main reason why I was packing on more belly fat.

Cortisol
A.K.A.
"Beer Belly Syndrome"

WARNING: Boring Science Stuff:
Cortisol is a stress hormone, it gets released during times when extreme pressure is put on your nervous system (e.g. running long distances).

What Cortisol does is tells your body to intentionally store fat, specifically in the mid-section.

It's a safety measure in case you keep piling on the pressure, and your blood sugar drops - causing you to pass out. Your body would have to eat that fat store just to keep you alive.

So the running wasn't doing what I thought it was doing...

My heart & lungs had never been stronger - which felt amazing - but my goal was to get a six pack, and I wasn't working towards that goal.

You see it in runners all the time.

They are putting their bodies through
extreme amounts of stress,
cortisol get's released into the mid-section,
and the more they run...
the more belly fat they have.

They may have skinny arms and legs
(I did, anyway)
but the belly fat is still there.

Also I was doing tons of crunches and ab-
work every day. The problem was - all that
was doing was building my ab muscles.

There was still a layer of fat on top of them,
so nobody could see them. (Talk about a
waste of time!)

I had confused fitness - which is great! - with
weight loss

When it comes to losing weight, you've got to stay focused on what's important...

It's all about looking good naked in front of the mirror

Let me go ahead and be blunt here: You want to look a certain way while standing in front of the mirror.

Let's call a spade a spade.

The politically correct thing to say is that *"losing weight is important for your health, your kidneys, your heart, your joints, and your longevity."*

And it is!
But that's not why you're reading this book.

You're reading this right now because you want your body to look a certain way.

Nothing more.

Ok, now that we got that outta the way, we can keep our focus on what you're after - losing weight in order to look a certain way in front of the mirror.

Losing Weight Made Easy

In a minute I'm going to tell you some methods and strategies to losing weight that will be 100% new to you. What I'm about to share with you is going to blow your mind for three main reasons.

1. It's completely backwards from what you've been told

2. Just how *SIMPLE* the process can be

   .....And

3. How quickly you can get results! <-- we've been conditioned to believe that we can, or should, only lose 2lbs per week. What you're about to learn is going to blow that method of thinking out of the water!

But first, let me give you a quick overview of weight loss and how it really works, so that when we get into the specifics, you truly grasp them.

Simply put, weight loss is a reversal process.

You've been doing something that caused your body to put on the weight, and now all we've got to do is pin-point what the cause is, and do the opposite!

I was listening to a speech one time, and the speaker said he would share the key to financial success with us.

"It's so simple," he exclaimed. "The Key to financial success is"….

"Observe what poor people do….
and then don't do that!"

I remember sitting there thinking *"WOW!! What a stupidly simple truth!"* And it's just as true for wealth as it is for weight loss.

The ONLY weight loss advice you'll ever need!
(The most simple method of losing fat)

Here's the secret to weight loss:

<u>"Observe what overweight people do....and then don't do that!"</u>

Do I need to say more?

Honestly, weight loss is more about reversing something you've done, than it is learning something new. (although I'm going to be sharing some really cool, new, exciting body-science tricks here shortly that will drastically speed-up the process!)

People who struggle to lose weight come up with all sorts of interesting rationales. I've heard people claim they can't lose weight for all kinds of reasons:

- *"My thyroid is messed up"*
- *"It's genetic"*
- *"I don't have time to exercise"*
- *"My meds cause me to retain weight"*
- *"It's my age"*

The funny thing, though, is that when I see the same people that make these types of excuses in the grocery line, the contents of their baskets are the <u>opposite</u> of what's in mine. It never fails.

Try this next time you're at the grocery store or a restaurant:

Start observing people in the checkout lines, take notice of what's in their basket. When you're out to eat, take notice of what's on the plate of the person one table over.

You'll start to notice a trend very quickly.

Observe the behaviors of what the average overweight person does, and then don't do it! Seriously, that's it!

So then the obvious next question is:

"What behavior was I doing that caused me to gain weight?"

A lot of people think that weight gain is caused by a lack of activity. *"Ugh, ever since I got this desk job I've put on 30lbs."*

But on a biochemical level, that has literally nothing to do with it.

Understand this:

The only reason you have fat on your body is because your body is protecting itself from YOU!

Fat is a safety feature built-in to your body. It builds-up to protect the body from a number of harmful things.

Fat doesn't accumulate because you have a desk job - there are plenty of lean people working in cubicles. Fat could care less where you spend your 9 - 5.

Your body also doesn't store fat because you ate too much fat. Roughly 75% of an Eskimo's diet is whale & seal blubber - and they are much leaner than the typical American.

(Sidenote: In 1977 the term 'Eskimo' was deamed inappropriate, but most people wouldn't recognize the term *Inuit*....so, I apologize to any Inuits I've offended)

Let me show you the 3 main reasons the body stores fat, and then you'll be able to see which one[s] caused *you* to gain weight. Then all we'll have to do to get rid of it is REVERSE the cause:

The 3 _MAIN_ Causes
of Weight Gain

Cause #1: To Protect Your Blood Sugar
Levels

This is hands-down the number one most prevalent cause of weight gain. Most likely, you could throw out all the others, focus on reversing this one, and you'd be set.

When you consume too much sugar, your body quickly rushes all of the excess sugar out of your bloodstream and into your fat stores. **I don't need to get any more technical than that**.

You're going to have the natural tendency to look at the other two causes of weight gain and focus on one of them because they're more complex, and sexier-sounding causes...

Don't even go there yet!

Until you've fixed problem #1...
<u>The others don't matter!</u>

This is THE main reason people gain weight, and can't lose it.

I speak with people all the time who go on calorie restrictive diets. They're barely eating anything, but what they are eating are foods that have a bunch of sugars (a.k.a. carbs) in them.

They're starving themselves all day every day, and they're left bewildered by the fact that they're not losing weight.

Sugar consumption is the reason.

The good news is -

<u>YOU DO NOT HAVE TO STOP EATING SUGAR,</u>
in order to reverse this process.

I'm going to show you a nifty little "body hack", that allows you to consume sugar strategically, and lose rapid weight. We'll discuss that in just a few.

Now your natural tendency is going to be to you to ask *"Well how much sugar should I be having?"*

We'll get into specifics a little later, but here's the important thing to keep in mind before even asking that question:

***Don't draw a line in the sand,
and expect not to flirt with it.***

If I tell you that you should not exceed 100g sugar per day (FYI: that's an arbitrary number, so don't even think about it!), then you're probably going to eat 99g of sugar per day. That's still not going to cut it.

So for now, just focus on sugar itself.

Rather than counting - just begin taking notice. The best way to do this is to start asking yourself *"Does what I'm about to eat have sugar (carbs) in it?"*

Going back to the Health VS Weight Loss concept
we were discussing earlier, another thing people love to
get fixated on is what ***type*** of sugar/carb are they supposed to be eating.

"What's better cane sugar or brown sugar?
enriched flour or whole grain?
sucrose or fructose?
white or wheat?"

<u>All of that is superfluous!</u>

It's a waste of time to focus on.
It's all sugar, and it's the #1 cause of weight gain.

Let's move on.

<u>Cause #2: To Protect Your Thyroid & Hormones</u>

This can actually be caused by numerous things: emotional stress, eating too many chemicals, over-exertion/under consumption, to name a few.

This could be a *really* long section
if we wanted to get into it.I could go into
detail about cortisol, leptin, epinephrine,
blah, blah, blah! - But there's no need to do
all that.

I'd spend a lot of time talking, you'd check
facebook on your phone real quick, then
scroll down the page to get to this:

If you put stress on your liver,
your fat-<u>burning</u> hormones will shut down,
AND
your fat-<u>storing</u> hormones will kick in!

Here's all you need to know...

Your daily habits are causing your hormones to get out-o-whack. But rather than trying to pick apart which specific behaviors are causing this, we'll just put a simple system in place to reverse ALL of it.

Sound good?

Perfect.

*BUT - keep in mind. Reversing this cause of weight gain, will only matter if you've fixed the first cause of weight gain: Blood Sugar.

Cause #3: To Protect Your Organs

Let's take a quick trip back to 7th grade science class for a second, and discuss pH balance.

Hang with me for one sec!

This isn't the most exciting topic in the world, but if you're looking to lose weight, you'll want to pay attention.

Your body is in a constant struggle to balance your pH levels ("pH" stands for Potential of Hydrogen...not important here).

It's important that you remain slightly alkaline in order to be functioning properly. But the foods you've been eating produce acid, which turns your blood very acidic.

When you constantly do this...

**Your body HAS TO quickly build-up fat
around your organs
so that the acid doesn't eat away at them.**

So, while this is going on, you could be running 3 miles every day and working out for an hour with your trainer, but your body still isn't going to get rid of that fat.

It *CAN'T*!
It's there to protect your organs from the acid.

The only way to get *that* fat off, is by eliminating the acid in your blood.

But don't get too caught-up on how to fix this right now.

The system you're about to learn is going to reverse this, without you even having to think about it!

Ok, now that you've learned the difference between heatlh & weight loss, and the 3 main reasons your body gains (and holds onto) weight, it's now time to reverse them...

Let's build your weight loss Strategy!

Weight Loss "How-To" Profile

How Joy Used this System to lose 15lbs in 2 weeks

Meet Joy.

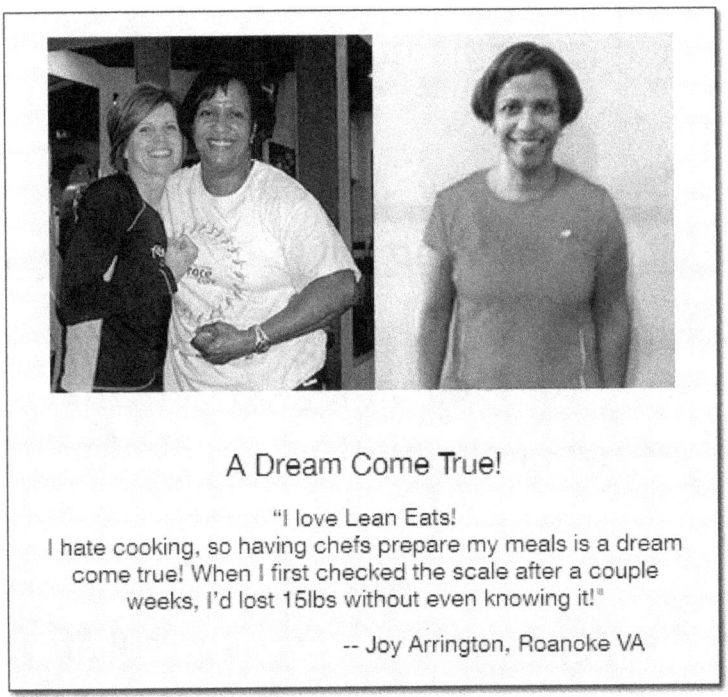

A Dream Come True!

"I love Lean Eats!
I hate cooking, so having chefs prepare my meals is a dream
come true! When I first checked the scale after a couple
weeks, I'd lost 15lbs without even knowing it!"

-- Joy Arrington, Roanoke VA

Joy had been working her butt of in the gym for months and the scale was barely budging...

She was obviously frustrated.

She was eating low calorie protein bars, drinking shakes, and stayed away from the soft drinks and snack foods.

She thought she was being pretty healthy...

But when joy implemented the strategies you're
about to read in the next section
(<u>especially the 3 step golden Weight Loss</u>
<u>Success Strategy</u>),
the weight started melting off of her faster than she ever imagined!

Now that Joy has learned the formula for weight loss
* <u>and just how simple it is</u> *
she is at her ideal weight, and loves the way she looks!
==================================

Section 2:

Building Your Weight Loss Strategy

Now I'm going to walk you through the process of weight loss. The beauty of this system is that it helps you counter all of the causes of weight gain - without having to dissect each one and attempting to reverse it.

I'll start by laying out the 3 part process, then we'll dive into each one more specifically.

1. **Carb Cycling Process**
   Carb cycling is a scientific way to regulate your blood sugar and manage your endocrine system.

2. **3 Step Golden Weight Loss Success Formula**

   This 3 step formula is the staple of the weight-loss process. It helps you streamline your weight loss regiment, and allows your results to become passive.

3. **Fat-burning Exercise Program (*Optional for best results)**

   You do not *have to* incorporate exercise for this system to work for you - but I highly recommend it. And this exercise system will go hand-in-hand with your carb cycling, and will allow you to get extremely rapid results.

Part 1:
Carb Cycling

How to Lose 20lbs in 28 Days

There are many different methods of carb cycling, but here are three primary ones that you can choose from to get started.

- Beginners Carb Cycle

- Advanced Carb cycle

- Keto Carb Cycle ← Extremely Rapid Results!!

Now I'm going to explain carb cycling real quick, so that when you see the difference in these methods, you'll understand what they mean.

So what *is* carb cycling?

Carb cycling is simply this: going through a period of low-carb consumption, followed by a period of high-carb consumption, back-and-forth in a cycle.

Strategies Produce Results

Here's why this works:
Each and every day, when you're exercising, walking around, or even sitting in a chair your body is burning carbs for energy.

Carbs are the quickest, most available source of energy – so it's the body's typical go-to. Fat is a much more powerful, efficient source of energy, so you're body would prefer to store it in case of emergency.

However with carb cycling, you're emptying your body's liver stores (carbs) so that it has to burn fat for energy.

If you cut out carbs all together (never recommended) then you're hormone levels drop and you eventually hit a plateau.

But by cycling your carbs, you help the body by speeding up the thyroid and raising your hormones to desirable levels (like a constant reset), so that your metabolism speeds up, and you can continue burning fat at a rapid rate.

Carb cycling also makes losing weight livable because you get a mental reset as well! You get to eat all of your favorite foods & drinks – and plenty of them – so that you don't ever feel deprived.

Alright, now that you understand a little bit more about how carb cycling works, let's take a look at the breakdown of the 3 different methods here.

	Day 1	Day 2	Day 3	Day 4	Day 5	Day 6	Day 7
Beginners Carb Cycle	Low Carb ⬇	⬆ High Carb	Low Carb ⬇	⬆ High Carb	Low Carb ⬇	⬆ High Carb	⬆ High Carb
Advanced Carb Cycle	Low Carb ⬇	No Carb ⬇	⬆ High Carb	Low Carb ⬇	No Carb ⬇	⬆ High Carb	⬆ High Carb
Keto Carb Cycle	Low Carb ⬇	Low Carb ⬇	Low Carb ⬇	Low Carb ⬇	Low Carb ⬇	Low Carb ⬇	⬆ High Carb

As you can see here, it's a strategy for weight loss (not a philosophy). It's a system you can run over and over again to get the results you want.

=====================================

Here's a short video where I talk about
how to use the keto carb cycle method
to lose 20lbs in just a few weeks!

www.myleaneats.com/#!video-lose-20lbs-in-28-days/czns

***This is the method you'll use to lose your
first 20lbs, then you'll switch to the next
level of carb cycling for maintenance.**

=====================================

On those low carb days, the body is depleting the carbs it has and it begins using fat for energy. Obviously the Keto Carb Cycle has the most opportunity for rapid fat-loss.

Here's how you can best use these methods:

It would seem obvious that you would want to start with the "beginners" carb cycle especially if you're new to it, and then progress to the more advanced methods.

But actually, the best way you can use this is by starting with the keto carb cycle, and progressively working your way backwards. Here's why...

In the beginning of a weight loss program, it's important to build momentum. Results wane, period. So, if you start off with slow results, you'll see less-and-less progress.

That's not the best way to start.

You want to start strong and get *GREAT* results from the beginning, then as you progress towards your ideal weight (or how you want to look in the mirror), you work into the methods that produce less rapid results.

And once you've reached your ideal weight, and you've seen how simple - and FUN! - carb cycling is, you'll want to use it for maintenance.

Maintaining Your Ideal Weight

At this point you might be wonder if you need to alter anything about carb cycling in order to maintain, once you've reached your goal.

Nope, the same method that's used to help you burn fat will also keep you at your ideal weight.

How can this be?

Because remember: weight loss is a reversal process. Carb cycling isn't doing something magical to your body. It's simply reversing all of the things you were doing to it before.

And as you stay on it, and those weight-gaining behaviors are eliminated, carb cycling will work to keep you where you are.

Pretty cool, right?

Ok, so now that you understand carb cycling and have decided on which method you're going to begin with, let's talk about the 3-Step Golden Weight Loss Strategy.

Part 2:
3-Step Golden Weight Loss Success Strategy

I call this the golden weight loss success strategy in hopes that the name will tell you just how powerful and important it is.

I can predict your weight loss results right here, right now

Every time I see someone beginning a weight loss program, I can predict right from the beginning whether they will be successful or not. And the way I do that is whether they use this 3 step strategy....or not.

I can honestly tell you that every success story I can think of, used this strategy. And every person I can think of that did NOT get the results they wanted, ignored this strategy, and tried to use the "cool new tricks" they just learned, with no rhyme or reason.

Don't kid yourself, lean people eat by a strategic plan.
This right here will determine your success.

Here's the 3 step formula (that I personally use every week) that will bring your carb cycling plan to life.

Step #1) **Have a plan**
Obviously you can't stick to a plan if you don't have one. The carb cycling chart is a plan, but it's not *YOUR* full plan.

You need to take a few minutes and map out exactly which meals you're going to eat, and at what times, on which days.

This shouldn't be complicated, and will only take you about 5 minutes to do.

Here's an example menu:

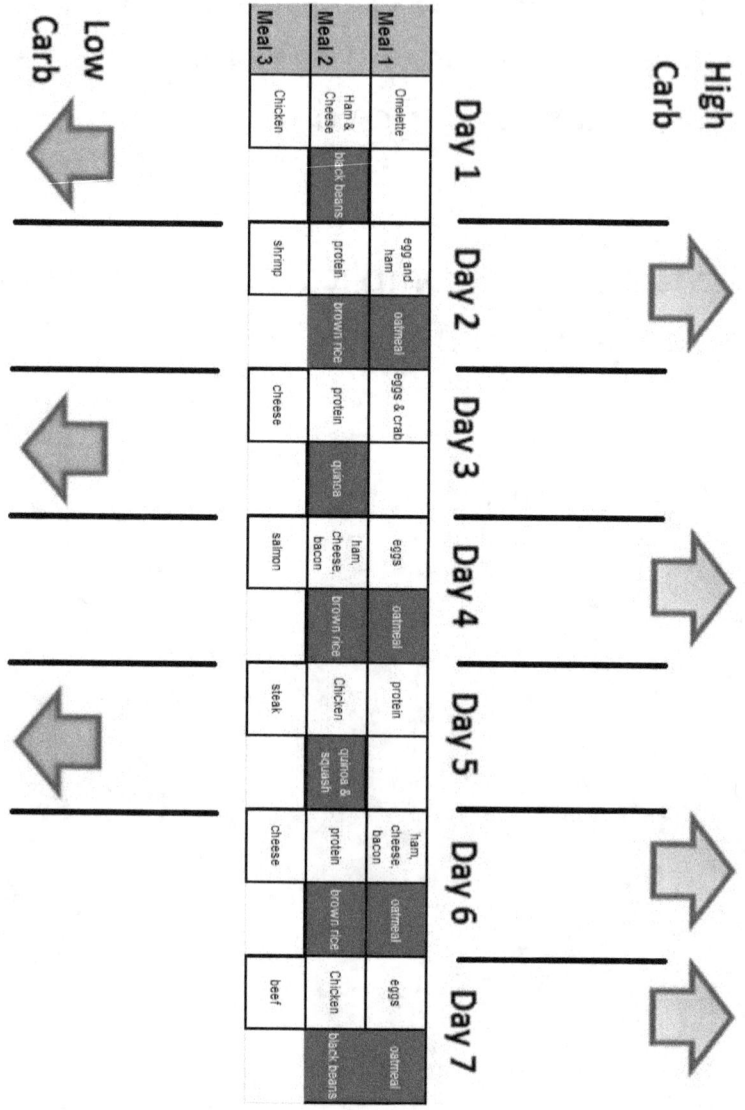

	Day 1	Day 2	Day 3	Day 4	Day 5	Day 6	Day 7
Meal 1	Omelette	egg and ham / oatmeal	eggs & crab	eggs / oatmeal	protein	ham, cheese, bacon / oatmeal	eggs / oatmeal
Meal 2	Ham & Cheese / black beans	protein / brown rice	protein / quinoa	ham, cheese, bacon / brown rice	Chicken / quinoa & squash	protein / brown rice	Chicken / black beans
Meal 3	Chicken	shrimp	cheese	salmon	steak	cheese	beef

High Carb

Low Carb

This is an example of the "beginner carb cycle". As you can see, every other day is a higher carb day.

The purples represent starches (full-blown carbs). Notice, there are two purples on the high carb days, and only one purple on the low carb days.

This is a powerful strategy for weight loss that will work extremely well.

But don't over-think the actual meals for now - that's a more advanced strategy for later. Just note that each meal is primarily protein based, and that you have fewer carbs on low carb days, and higher carbs on high carb days - simple.

Now let's take the exact same menu, and alter it towards the "keto carb cycle" strategy.

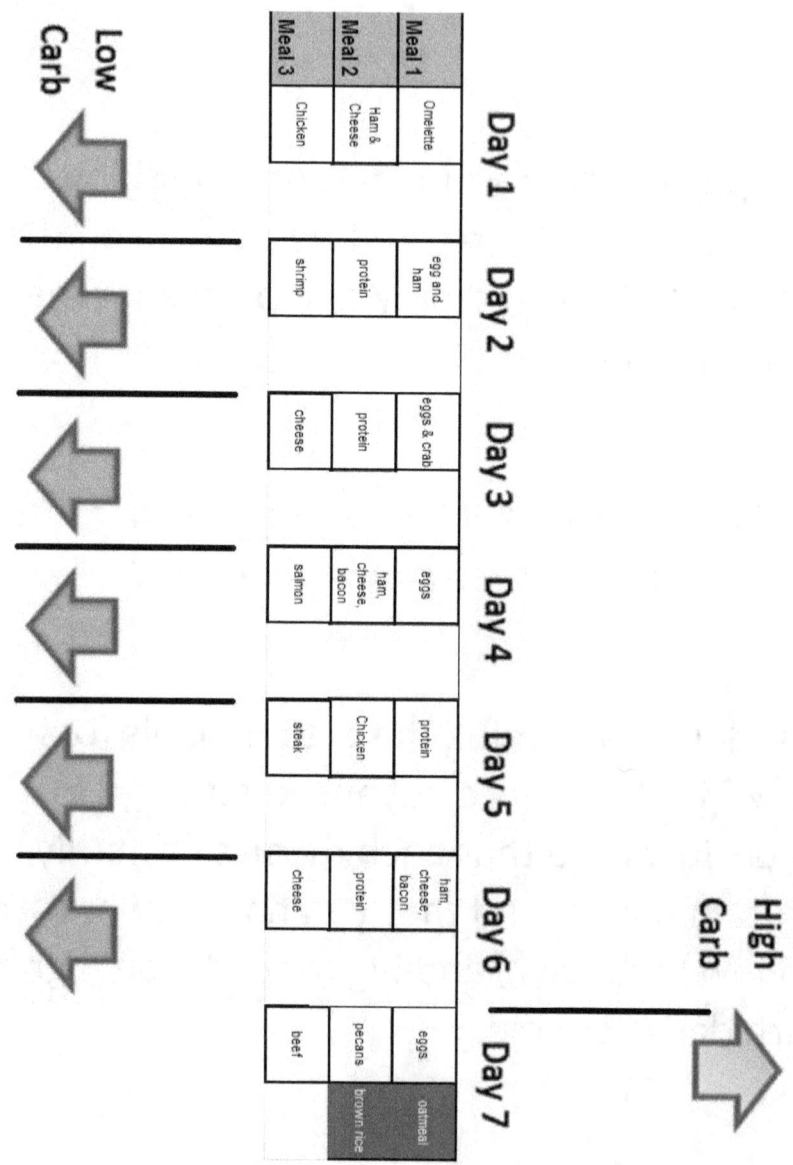

	Day 1	Day 2	Day 3	Day 4	Day 5	Day 6	Day 7	
High Carb →
Meal 1	Omelette	egg and ham	eggs & crab	eggs	protein	ham, cheese, bacon	eggs	oatmeal
Meal 2	Ham & Cheese	protein	protein	ham, cheese, bacon	Chicken	protein	pecans	brown rice
Meal 3	Chicken	shrimp	cheese	salmon	steak	cheese	beef	
← Low Carb

Notice here that we took out all of the purples (carbs) except for on the one high carb day.

When using the "keto carb cycle" strategy, it works best to go more to the extreme by taking out the starches on the low carb days. In reality there are still carbs on those days - for example the beef may be a meatloaf (which has carbs), or the protein may have oatmeal in it - but it helps to keep your carbs extremely low for this strategy.

The important thing about this step is just to choose your meals.
Don't worry about being specific yet...
just pick them.

If you end up going out to a restaurant for dinner, for example, on Day 5, you know you're going to have steak. Doesn't necessarily matter how it's prepared...just have some kind of steak.

Also, don't get caught-up on the number of meals per day. I use three as a general example, but if you normally eat 5, 6 ,7 meals each day that's fine. (And I'm also referring to "snacks" as meals)

So, if you get home after the restaurant and are still hungry, but you've eaten your three meals, no problem. Have another protein. This won't affect the high/low carb day strategy.

Starting to make sense?

Bottom line:
Have a plan (written or typed) print it out, and keep it somewhere you can refer to it often.

Step #2)   **<u>Have your meals prepared in advance</u>**

This is the step that determines your success possibly more than anything else in this book.

The decision you make right here - to prepare, or not to prepare - will define your results.

The reason this is such an incredibly important step is because when you're busy, you don't have time to think about what to eat next. Even if you've got your gameplan ready, and you want to follow it, <u>if the meals aren't readily-available, you WILL veer off of your plan</u>.

This doesn't have to be complicated, and it doesn't have to be 100% in order to work.

You may go out to eat 2 nights/week, so no need to prepare those meals in advance. Maybe Saturday & Sunday the family cooks dinner together - that's two more meals you don't have to worry about for now.

But it's important to have roughly 80% of your meals cooked, portioned, and put into separate containers. This will be a life-saver once the week starts.

If you don't have the time to do this, or are overwhelmed at the thought of it, or if you simply have no clue where to begin...

```
==========================
```
Insert Blatant Advertisement
```
==========================
```

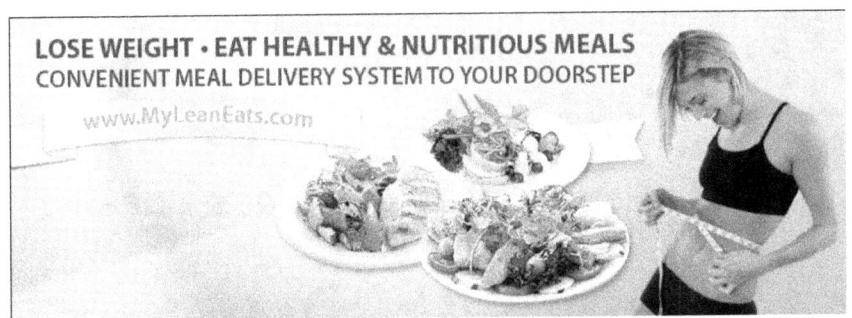

Lean Eats *can* do all of this work for you.

The chefs will:

- Buy your groceries

- Cook & portion all of your meals

- Cut your meals like chicken into bite-size pieces (in case you have to eat-on-the-go)

- They'll even put a color sticker on each meal (<u>so you know when to eat each meal</u>)

- ***AND they will do it for less $$ than you can do it yourself!! ← *That's* a deal!

AND, since you're reading this book, you can get a 1-time 15% off Coupon Code for your first order.

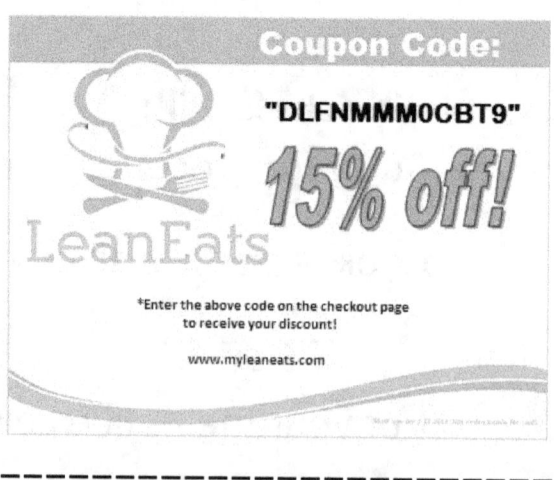

========================

End of Blatant Advertisement

========================

Remember....

This is possibly the most important step of your weight loss strategy!

Regardless of whether you have the chefs prepare your meals for you, or if you prepare them on your own, <u>they need to be in your fridge before you begin the first day</u>.

Step #3)   **<u>Put your meals in order</u>**

It would be very easy to overlook this step as being redundant. But let me tell you that this step brings step #2 to life.

Ok, so you're meals are prepared and sitting in your fridge, but when you're scrambling to get out the door, and you have to sort through and find your specific meals for the day, this step makes *ALL* the difference.

This takes no time at all,
and saves you all the time in the world.

Start with your day 7 meals, put them at the back of the fridge. Then your work your way backwards to day 1 - which should end-up in the very front of the fridge.

A pretty simple step.

As you'll see, the beauty of this 3 step formula is that it will make weight loss passive throughout the week. You just grab the next meal, eat it, and don't think about it.

The next thing you know, you'll hop on the scale after day 7, and you've lost 7lbs!!

That's pretty darn cool :)

Now let's talk about the exercise part of your weight loss strategy.

Part 3:
Fat-burning Exercise Program

Like I said before, you do not *have to* incorporate exercise for this system to work for you - but I highly recommend it. And this exercise system will go hand-in-hand with your carb cycling, which will allow you to get extremely rapid results.

(Disclaimer: If you're currently working with a coach or trainer, do NOT veer off of the plan they have designed for you. I would start by telling them that you're thinking about starting a carb cycling routine, and would like to know if it will go hand-in-hand with the current program they have you on.)

So real quick, let me show you the different types of exercise, what they're for, and then show you how to choose the right ones for your weight loss strategy.

- **<u>Hypertrophy</u>**
  This is what fitness models and bodybuilders do. It's very slow, it involves lifting heavy weights, and the sole intention is aesthetics. This style of exercise simply builds your muscles bigger.

- **Endurance Training**

  This is what marathon runners do. It's very repetitive, it's not intense at all, and requires minimal - if any - heavy lifting. The intention here is typically sports performance such as marathons and triathlons. This style of exercise builds your slow twitch muscle fibers, and your capillaries for extended periods of blood flow.

- **Power Training**

  This is what Olympic athletes, CrossFitters and football players do. It's very active, extremely intense, and typically involves heavy weights. The intention is typically nothing more than to get more powerful at the exercise you're performing. This style of exercise builds your neuromechanics and your fast twitch muscle fibers.

- **<u>Metabolic Conditioning</u>** (often confused with Power Training)
  This is what fitness models, supermodels, and people wanting to lose weight do. It's intense yet done in strategic intervals, it is designed around heart rate, and sometimes involves weights - but not always. The intention here is to speed up your metabolism and burn fat.

- **<u>Cardio</u>** (often confused with endurance training)
  Just about everyone does this in one form or another - either walking, jogging or anything slow - moderate and rhythmic. The intention here is to improve heart, lungs and bloodflow, and very often extra fat-burning.

- **General Fitness**

  This is what beginners, fitness enthusiasts, the elderly and the average person just wanting to remain "fit" do. It can be anything from pilates to core exercise, general weight-training to yoga, and more. It's good for numerous things such as for people just trying to remain active, or the prevention of osteoporosis. It can be used to develop flexibility, core strength, blood flow, or even relaxation.

Ok now that you've got a basic overview of the different types of exercise, let's pick which ones you're going to use, and plug them into your strategy. (Again, ask your coach or trainer before attempting to make any changes to your current routine)

	Hypertrophy	Endurance Training	Power Training	Metabolic Training	Cardio	General Fitness
Used for Strategic Weight loss	✓			✓	✓	

These are the 3 primary types of exercise that best aid weight loss.

*Hypertrophy isn't typically associated with weight loss.

But it is designed to increase muscle mass.

(that toned look)

And the more muscle you have in your legs, arms, etc., the more fat your body burns all day long.

Now this doesn't mean you can't use the other types of exercise on the chart - and of course many types of exercise are hybrids of many of these. You may be training for an event, or just love doing CrossFit, for example. That's ok too!

The important thing here is to use fat-burning exercise
as your foundation,
and any other types of exercise
as recreation.

It's important to understand the difference between the various types of exercise - this will allow you to reach your goal quicker, and avoid frustration from overworking yourself with little results.

It's very common for people to confuse cardio with endurance training.

Visualize a young man or woman who is trying to burn-off their belly fat, going crazy on an Eliptical machine, legs burning, shirt soaked.

Endurance training doesn't typically burn fat from the body (remember my example earlier about marathon runners having belly fat), so this person is destined to be frustrated because they'll keep working hard, and wondering why they don't see a difference in their body.
This is why it's so important to understand the different types of exercise, and pick the ones that will yield the best results for your weight loss strategy.

Here are 3 different weight-loss exercise regimens you can choose from to get started.

Exercise Strategy #1: Rapid Weight Loss

As the name implies, this exercise strategy is designed for the most rapid weight-loss.

It works well for beginners as it doesn't yet include Hypertrophy training which is slightly more advanced.

Day 1	Day 2	Day 3	Day 4	Day 5	Day 6	Day 7
Metabolic Training	Cardio	Metabolic Training	Cardio	Metabolic Training	Cardio	Rest
Exp: High Intensity Interval Training	Exp: Walking, light jogging	Exp: High Intensity Interval Training	Exp: Walking, light jogging	Exp: High Intensity Interval Training	Exp: Walking, light jogging	

In case you're new to exercising, don't let the looks of this regimen intimidate you.

The metabolic training can take as few as 15 - 20 minutes to do, and the cardio you're probably already doing to an extent.

It's pretty basic, straight forward, and doesn't require a lot of knowledge about these types of exercise in order to begin.

And I've made it **EASY** for you!

If you want to learn the fundamentals of metabolic training, and for a done-for-you program that you can follow right away...

Here is a FREE video series on the quick ends-and-outs of metabolic training. (rbt.infusionsoft.com/go/mrtsq/LE/)

Discover How and Why Metabolic Resistance Training will Triple YOUR Rapid Fat Loss Results

And don't worry - it's 100% FREE.

Grab it now, before you forget, because this goes hand-in-hand with your carb cycling strategy,
and it will *DRASTICALY* speed-up your weight loss results.

(rbt.infusionsoft.com/go/mrtsq/LE/)

Exercise Strategy #2: Burn Fat / Build Muscle

This strategy is a great plateau breaker.

It's a slightly more advanced strategy, and I don't recommend beginning Hypertrophy training without consulting your coach or trainer first.

With this strategy you begin using all 3 different types of fat-burning exercise methods - and you begin to notice some muscle tone too.

Day 1	Day 2	Day 3	Day 4	Day 5	Day 6	Day 7
Metabolic Training	Cardio	Hypertrophy	Metabolic Training	Cardio	Hypertrophy	
Exp: High Intensity Interval Training	Exp: Walking, light jogging	Exp: Weight Training	Exp: High Intensity Interval Training	Exp: Walking, light jogging	Exp: Weight Training	Rest

Exercise Strategy #3: Getting Toned

This strategy cuts back a little bit on the cardio, and works a little more into a maintenance regimen.

By the time you're ready to begin this type of strategy, you should be well on your way to approaching your goal weight.

Day 1	Day 2	Day 3	Day 4	Day 5	Day 6	Day 7
Metabolic Training	Hypertrophy	Metabolic Training	Hypertrophy	Metabolic Training	Hypertrophy	Cardio
Exp: High Intensity Interval Training	Exp: Weight Training	Exp: High Intensity Interval Training	Exp: Weight Training	Exp: High Intensity Interval Training	Exp: Weight Training	Exp: Walking, light jogging

You can use any variation of these exercise regimens - and of course, if you're new to exercise, you may want to simply start by doing cardio (walking or light jogging) 3 days per week.

Now We'll Put it All Together

Now I'm going to take each of the exercise strategies, and match them to the carb cycling strategies that you learned earlier.

Full Strategy #1

If you're just starting out, this is the strategy I would recommend for you.

This yields the most rapid weight loss, and is really easy to get started.

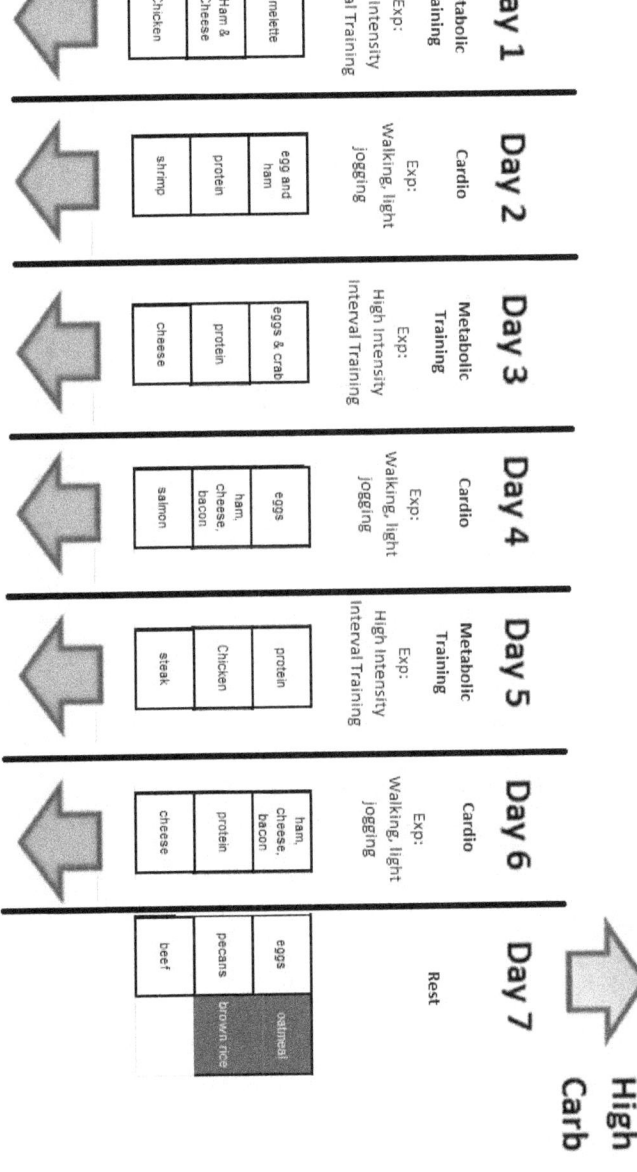

	Day 1	Day 2	Day 3	Day 4	Day 5	Day 6	Day 7
Exercise	Metabolic Training Exp: High Intensity Interval Training	Cardio Exp: Walking, light jogging	Metabolic Training Exp: High Intensity Interval Training	Cardio Exp: Walking, light jogging	Metabolic Training Exp: High Intensity Interval Training	Cardio Exp: Walking, light jogging	Rest
Meal 1	Omelette	egg and ham	eggs & crab	eggs	protein	ham, cheese, bacon	eggs oatmeal
Meal 2	Ham & Cheese	protein	protein	ham, cheese, bacon	Chicken	protein	pecans brown rice
Meal 3	Chicken	shrimp	cheese	salmon	steak	cheese	beef

Low Carb ← ... → **High Carb**

Remember: if this looks like too much to begin all at once, just start with the eating strategy, and come back to the exercise once you've got the eating mastered.

Full Strategy #2

Once you've seen some good results for a couple of weeks from using the first strategy - you would then want to wean yourself into this one.

It's a little less extreme, and it will get you to start building some muscle.

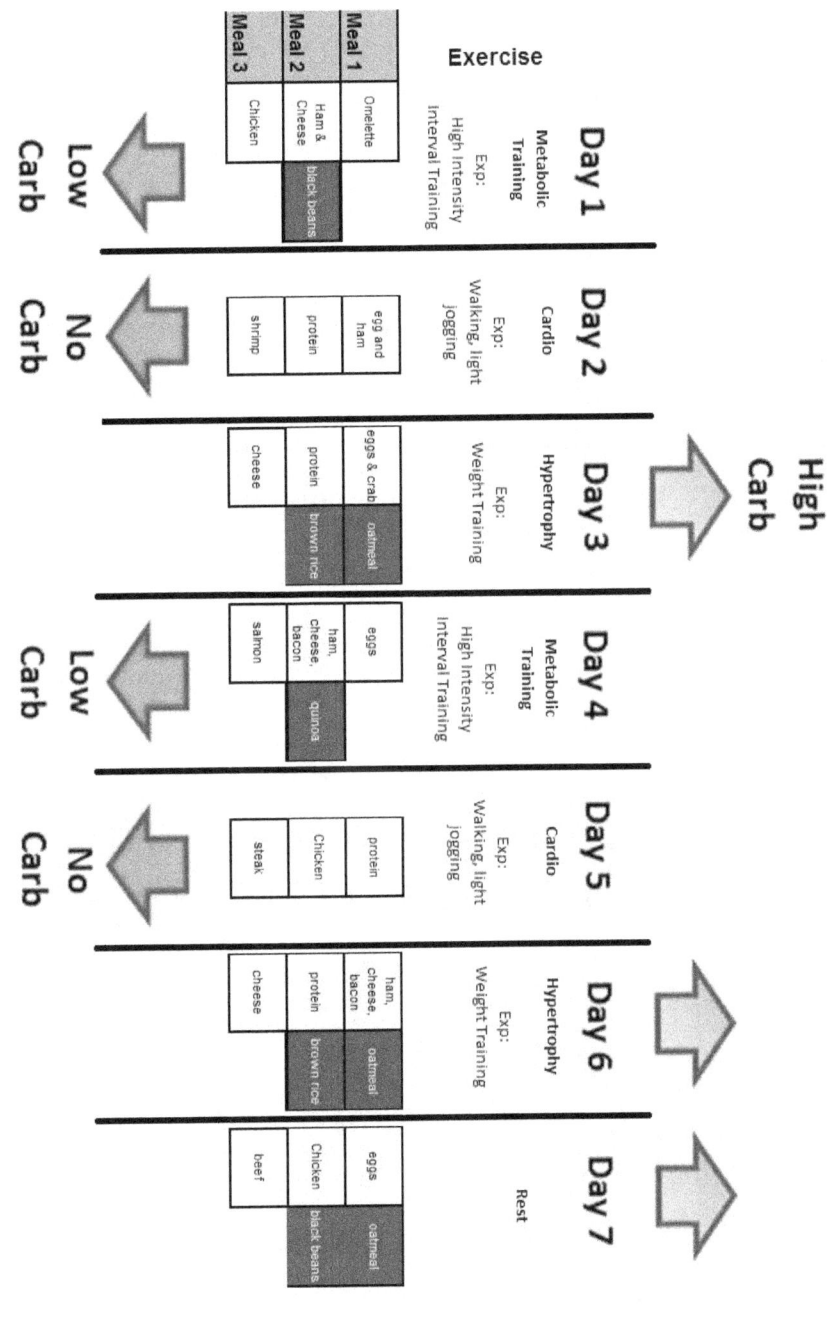

	Day 1	Day 2	Day 3	Day 4	Day 5	Day 6	Day 7
Exercise	Metabolic Training	Cardio	Hypertrophy	Metabolic Training	Cardio	Hypertrophy	Rest
	Exp: High Intensity Interval Training	Exp: Walking, light jogging	Exp: Weight Training	Exp: High Intensity Interval Training	Exp: Walking, light jogging	Exp: Weight Training	
Meal 1	Omelette / black beans	egg and ham	eggs & crab / oatmeal	eggs / quinoa	protein	ham, cheese, bacon / oatmeal	eggs / oatmeal
Meal 2	Ham & Cheese	protein	protein / brown rice	ham, cheese, bacon	Chicken	protein / brown rice	Chicken / black beans
Meal 3	Chicken	shrimp	cheese	salmon	steak	cheese	beef
	Low Carb	No Carb	High Carb	Low Carb	No Carb		

Since this strategy requires a change every single day, this takes a little more planning in advance.

You don't want to get caught trying to grab meals on the fly. So as you move into this strategy I'm going to stress how important it is to use the '3 Step Golden Weight Loss Success Strategy'.

If you're plan isn't written-down, prepared in advance, and organized in your fridge, this strategy becomes next to impossible to keep up with.

Again, don't get overwhelmed when thinking about all of this. Just go back, read through the preparation part, and set some time aside this weekend to do it.

Full Strategy #3

This strategy eases-up a little bit. It combines a maintenance exercise regimen with a liveable, on-going eating strategy to go along with it.

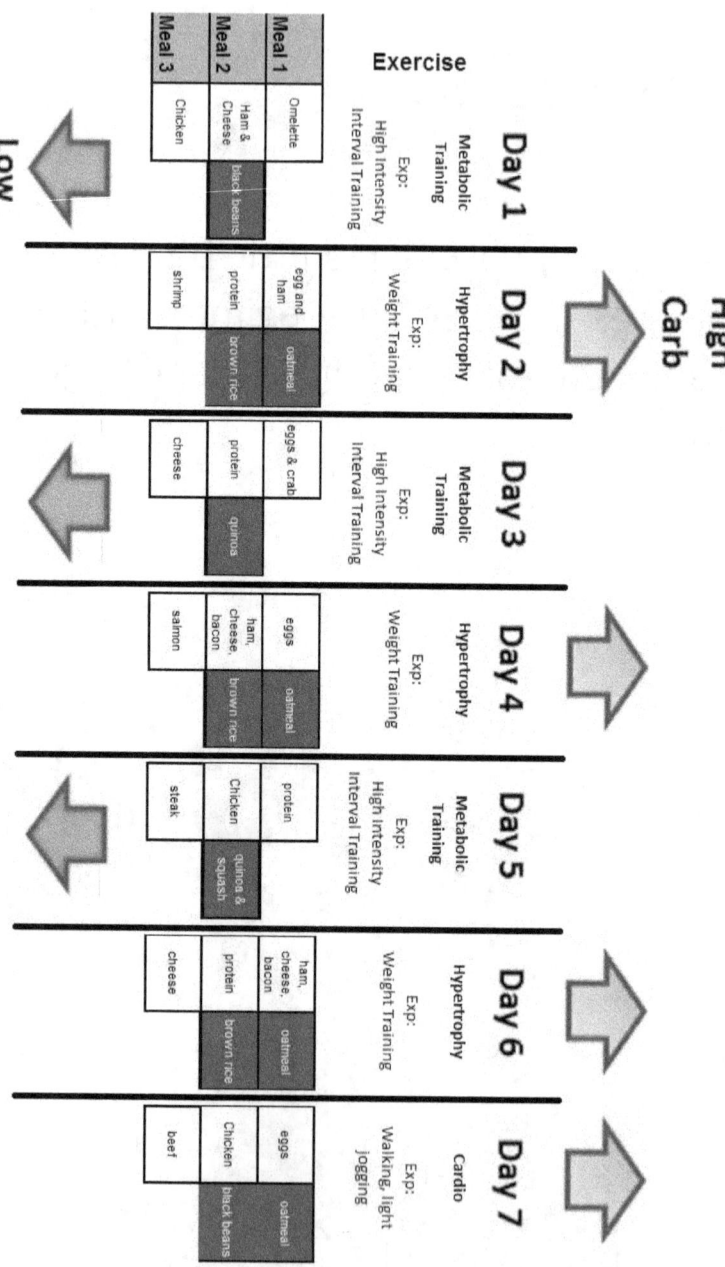

High Carb ← → **Low Carb**

	Day 1	**Day 2**	**Day 3**	**Day 4**	**Day 5**	**Day 6**	**Day 7**
Exercise	Exp: Metabolic Training / High Intensity Interval Training	Exp: Hypertrophy Weight Training	Exp: Metabolic Training / High Intensity Interval Training	Exp: Hypertrophy Weight Training	Exp: Metabolic Training / High Intensity Interval Training	Exp: Hypertrophy Weight Training	Exp: Cardio / Walking, light jogging
Meal 1	Omelette black beans	egg and ham / oatmeal	eggs & crab / quinoa	eggs / oatmeal	protein / quinoa & squash	ham, cheese, bacon / oatmeal	eggs / oatmeal
Meal 2	Ham & Cheese	protein / brown rice	protein	ham, cheese, bacon / brown rice	Chicken	protein / brown rice	Chicken / black beans
Meal 3	Chicken	shrimp	cheese	salmon	steak	cheese	beef

This is the typical type of regimen you would want to form as your on-going habit.

Does it have to be *EXACTLY* like this day-to-day, week-to-week?? No.

But ideally, if you stick to this basic strategy, you will stay weighing, looking, and feeling the way you want to - without having to think about it!

I can't tell you how life-changing it was to get in the habit of living by a strategy like this, and being able to spend my time thinking about other things, and yet still looking exactly the way I wanted to!

You're going to love it too.

Weight Loss "How-To" Profile

How Rick lost 140lbs!!

Meet Rick.

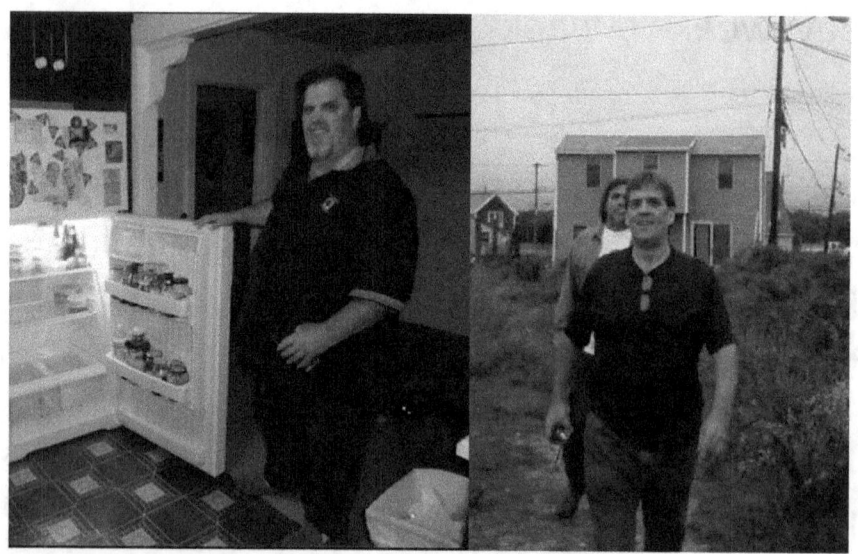

Rick was a pizza lover – a weight loss program was out of the question to him because he thought he'd have to give his pizza up.

One day I asked Rick "What if I told you, you could eat pizza every day, for an entire week, and lose 7lbs?"

Needless to say, he was suspicious...

He decided he'd start off by doing the Keto Carb cycle for a week.
I sent him 21 servings of Lean Eats low-carb pizza, so that he could eat it 3 times a day if he wanted...and he did.

Well, he didn't lose 7lbs that first week....he ended-up losing 8lbs!

And soon he was able to move to the more advanced version of the carb cycle, where he was even eating "real" pizza on his high carb days, and *still* losing weight!

After roughly 6 months of strategic eating – and while still enjoying plenty of his favorite pizza – **Rick lost 140lbs, and didn't have to give up a single thing!**

Section 3:

Advanced Weight Loss Secrets

*Quick Disclaimer
These are powerful techniques that are typically used by individuals who have been exercising and dieting for years. It is recommended that you check with your doctor or certified nutrition advisor before implementing most of the techniques listed below.

You're going to love this section - because these are some pretty powerful & effective tricks you can start using right away!

But it's important to <u>remember that if you use any of these, without having & implementing an overall strategy, then any success you might have from them will be short-lived</u>.

That being said, it's now time to dive in and put these secrets to work for you!

Fitness Model SECRET

Eat as much pizza as you want and burn fat

So if you want your cake...pizza...cookies...mexican food...ice cream, but still want to look lean & toned, I've got the secret you've been waiting for.

A lot of fitness models know & use this, but of course they don't necessarily want everyone else knowing it!.

The SECRET:
Your body cannot burn fat & store it at the same time.

So here's how to put this to use:
You eat your favorite cheat food, then you do some sort of moderate activity (cardio exercise) that gets your body burning fat WHILE you're digesting the food.

This way none of the calories consumed can actually make it into your fat stores—instead they circulate in the blood and get used for energy.

As hard as it is to believe, _the key to the whole trick is to do "moderate" activity_.

Anything too intense and your body stops burning fat,
and starts burning carbs
...which means it can still store fat!

Body Builder SECRET

Use Ice Cream to burn fat

Yep, you read it right!

Some of the old-school bodybuilders made this popular. They used to eat ice cream everyday as one of their methods for burning fat & building muscle.

No, not some kind of zero sugar ice cream....the good stuff!

But it isn't the ice cream, specifically, that makes this work. <u>They're using a trick called carb back-loading</u>.

The Science (in a nutshell)

First, this trick works only right after an intense bout of exercise. I'm talking about the ones where you are completely drained, your muscles have become useless, and you have to crawl out of the gym.

Immediately upon completing the workout, what happens is your liver & muscle stores have been depleted of their energy sources (i.e. sugar).

Your body will spend roughly the next hour scrambling to pull from other areas to make up for this sugar-drought. So you can do your body a favor...

Give it what it wants!

If you give it a simple sugar (ice cream) during this period, it absorbs it right up, and doesn't let your fat stores have any of it!

Carb <u>Back</u>-Loading

So that ice cream, or bread, or *WHATEVER* you decide to use, will actually help your body!

Type of Exercise
Remember you can't spend 60 minutes on the elliptical machine, and think because you're drained and exhausted that you've exercised enough to be able to utilize this trick.

Sorry!

This will only work if you've actually torn down your muscle fibers during exercise. That means you've got to be going intense! (Hypertrophy training works best for this)

I hear you, you're legs were burning on the elliptical

But here's how it works:
Anything that you can do for 30 minutes strait, just isn't intense enough for this rule to work.

Workout hard - tear your muslces - eat some ice cream :)

Hormone SECRET

Carb Loading

This is different than carb <u>back</u>-loading, which was the ice cream trick.

Here's how to do it
At the end of a carb cycle (think Keto Carb Cycle from section 2), you'll intentionally eat abundance of carbohydrates: Pasta, bread, chips, sandwiches......like a "cheat meal".

Here's why this works
During a week of low carbs, the body's hormone levels drop, and the thyroid (which dictates your metabolism) slows down.

When these things happen, your body stops yielding fat-burning results. <u>This is why people who do a low-carb diet long term, hit plateaus</u>.

By using a carb-load in your strategy **you'll keep your fat-burning hormone levels buzzing** as you begin another carb cycle week.

Busy Person SECRET

Do NOT Eat Every 3 Hours

If you're a busy, on-the-go type of person with more items on your to-do list than there are hours in the month, this secret is definitely for you!

(*This also works well for people who travel a lot)

This is a neat little trick called Intermittent Fasting, or I.F. in the fitness realm.

Instead of eating every 3 hours, you strategically go for an extended period of time where you eat nothing at all. Then you squeeze a larger amount of food into a smaller window of time.

A Few Examples:

- <u>20/4 Method</u>:
  This is by far the most powerful method.

Here's an example of how you can use it: Stop eating dinner at 9pm on a given night. The next day have nothing but water all day long. Then at 5pm eat! Stop eating again at 9pm.

(20 hours of fasting, 4 hours of eating)

- <u>16/8 Method</u>:
  This method is a little easier for beginners of I.F., and it still works really well.

Here's an exmaple of how to use it:
Wake up first thing (6am'ish) and begin eating. Continue snacking and eating meals through the day until around 2pm. Then stop and don't eat anything else until the next morning!

(16 hours of fasting, 8 hours of eating)

The important thing to remember for <u>this trick to work is that you can't do anything to interrupt the fasting</u>.

If you have even a tiny snack during the fast, this weight loss trick will not work the way it's designed to.

6 pack abs Secret

The truth about getting a flat stomach

Let me just start off by saying, you've got abs. Trust me, they're down there.

You wouldn't have the ability to get out of bed if they weren't.
People like to think you get abs by doing ab exercises, but all that's really doing is building the hidden muscles that nobody can see.

Think about a guy trying to make his arms huge. He's going to work his biceps and triceps to make the muscles bigger - not smaller.

But it's not the lack of abs that's the reason you can't see them - it's 1 of 3 things on top of them.

1. Fat ← this will be taken care of by the strategy you're putting in place

   ...Then, once you get lean, there are two other reasons you'll have to address...

2. Water:
   When your sodium to water ratio is off, your body will store water in your fat cells.

   The trick to solve this is to manipulate the ratio. Cut back on your sodium, and drink more water.

FYI: don't guess. The exact amounts will change person-to-person. But If you're going to start drinking 100oz/day, get a jug and measure, otherwise you're just hoping.

3. Chemicals:
   When you eat processed foods - specifically, meals that a machine put together by pulling nutrients from other sources - your body struggles to digest them and sends the chemicals into your fat cells.

   Stop eating things like bars, and R.T.D. shakes (Ready-to-Drink shakes), and watch how quickly your ab muscles start to appear!

Super Keto

How I lost 10lbs in 1 week

If you're doing the keto carb cycle, here's a cool little trick that will take it your results to the next level.

You're going to strategically have higher fat content at the beginning of your week, and then almost no fat content the 2nd of.

At the same time, on your high fat days, you'll consume twice the amount of water you normally drink. And on the no fat days, you'll drop down to half of your normal levels.

Here's an example of what this might look like:

Monday – Wednesday

Eat high fat protein sources (egg yolks, salmon, chicken, beef, peanut butter, cheeses).

Drink 1 gallon and a half of water each day.

Thursday – Saturday

Low fat proteins sources (tuna, turkey breast, tilapia, egg whites, whey protein, low-fat cottage cheese).
Drink half a gallon or less of water each day.

And on Sunday you'll do a 20 hour fast (like mentioned in the "Busy Person Secrets" section) before carb loading. And around 5pm you'll do a carb load (as mentioned in the "Hormone Secret" section)

This yields some really quick results, <u>but I wouldn't recommend it for beginners</u>. Only after you're very familiar with the keto carb cycle, and have used it successfully, would I attempt this strategy.

Alcohol SECRET
How to have a social life
...while losing weight

If you can give up your wine (or beer...or liquor) for a few weeks or months until you reach your goal weight—go for it!

BUT, since we know that's probably not going to happen, I figured I might as well let you in on a few really cool tricks you can use to keep losing weight WHILE drinking!

<u>First of all, the important thing to know here is that alcohol is sugar!</u>
<u>And sugar is bad (for weight loss)</u>.

Now that we know that, all we have to do is trick our body into needing sugar, so that it can't be stored as fat. You've got two different options for this:

Option 1 (recommended for nightly "Social-lites")

About 15 – 20 minutes prior to your first drink, you want to perform roughly 10 – 15 minutes of Metabolic Training (specifically, HIIT, a.k.a. High Intensity Interval Training).

What is this?

It's when you go-all-out and exert yourself 100% for a very short period—60 or so seconds. Then you rest for 30 seconds, and repeat for 10 – 15 minutes. Examples of activities you could do would be sprinting, hitting a punching bag, jumping jacks, or burpees.

What does this do?

It exhausts and opens up your liver & muscle stores to desperately need sugars.

So a few minutes after you finish, when you consume your drink, your liver & muscles soak every bit up, and your fat stores remain untouched!

Option 2 (recommended for those who are willing to go 5 – 6 nights without drinking) You're going to go through the entire week on a low-carb diet (and of course without drinking). You're going to save up your drinks for Saturday. (Same as Carb Loading)

Then when the weekend hits, you're going....."enjoy" yourself (wink-wink). I'm not saying you should overdo it—I'm saying, get it out of your system!

Check it out Here

rbt.infusionsoft.com/go/mrtsq/LE/

Macro Secret:

Calculating the exact amount
of food for you

In beginning your weight loss strategy, you don't have to worry about how much food you're eating. You'll get the same results regardless, and you'd just be spending a ton of time trying to keep track of one more thing!

This trick is for when you get closer and closer to your goal weight.

There are many different ways of going about this, but here's a general guideline you can use:

1. **Protein:**

    On average women want to multiply their goal weight by .9 (men by 1.2) to figure out how many grams they need per day.

    Example: if you want to weigh 120lbs, that's 120 x .9 = 108 grams of protein per day)

2. **Carbs:**

    Women want to multiply their goal weight by .4 (men by .6) to figure out how many grams they need per day.

    Example: if you want to weigh 120lbs, that's 120 x .4 = 48 grams of carbs per day)

Water:

To keep it simple, women & men can multiply their <u>BODY</u> weight by .9 to figure out how many ounces they need per day.

Example: if you currently weigh 140lbs, that's 140 x .9 = 126 ounces per day. That's basically a gallon.

*Note: Fat is an important macro-nutrient to
consider as well. But for our purposes here,
if you control these 3,
the fat will fall into place as it should!

You then take those 3 numbers, and divide them by how many meals you eat during the day—like this: Let's say you eat 5 meals each day.

1)   108g / 5 meals = 21 grams of protein per meal

2)   48g / 5 meals = 9 grams of carbs per meal

3)   126oz = Simply fill a gallon jug in the morning,

     and make sure it's empty before you go to bed!

Secret of Proximity

How to lose weight without trying...seriously!

Have you ever heard the saying: *"you are the average of the sum of the 5 people you spend the most time around?"*

This means if your 5 closest friends are wealthy, you'll soon become wealthy. If they're lazy, then you're either lazy or moving in that direction.

If the 5 people you spend the most time around are extremely lean...

then you will become more lean.

No matter how much we love sweets, or fast-food, or being lazy, <u>the fact of the matter is we are ALL influenced by those around us</u>. We adopt some of their behaviors without knowing it.

So if you want to start passively losing weight, one of the absolute smartest things you can do is to surround yourself with fit, lean people—people that who aspire to be like.

The ultimate secret to motivation

One of the top 2 – 3 difference between successful people and unsuccessful people is motivation.

Motivation is what separates those living their dream, from those who haven't quite made it yet. But not in the way you think….

People are always looking to find a way they can stay motivated, so that they'll keep working to achieve their goals.

Well, here's the secret to motivation…

Motivation is B.S.!

Just like you, those lean, front-of-a-magazine-cover people wake up some days and don't feel energized to do ANYthing!

So then how do they do it?

Understand that most people are constantly seeking motivation. They try to pump themselves up with a song or a video, or a mental state that urges them to get up and start **Do'ing**.

Conversely, successful people don't rely on motivation. They do the thing that needs to be done regardless of how they *feel*.

They could be bored, they could be tired, their attention could be temporarily drawn to something more compelling.....doesn't matter. They consistently do what needs to be done!

Here's how...

You've got to create a <u>Success System</u> to keep you on track when you're not motivated.

A friend of mine used to struggle getting her exercise in after a long day at work.

It wasn't that she hated exercise, the real struggle was getting herself motivated to go to the gym. That's the toughest part, when you're tired at the end of a long day, sometimes you just want to kick your feet up.

So here's how my friend designed a **Success System** to defeat her lack of motivation.

Every morning on her way to work, she would drive by her gym, and place her house key in a locker. Then after a long day at work, when she's exhausted mentally & physically, her natural desire was to go home and grab a glass of wine.

Well, the Success System she created for herself made it so that if she wanted to get into her house—she had to go by the gym.

Since the biggest struggle was always getting into the gym, **she found a way to win**!

She'd grab her key, be standing inside the locker room, and think to herself "well I'm already here....I might as well get on the treadmill for 10 min." And before she knew it, she had completed a 30 minute workout.

And that's the magic right there, <u>ignore motivation, and design a Success System to get yourself to stick to the plan regardless of how you *feel*</u>.

Weight Loss "How-To" Profile

How Ronda Lost Over 40lbs

Meet Ronda…. (I typically call her "Mom")

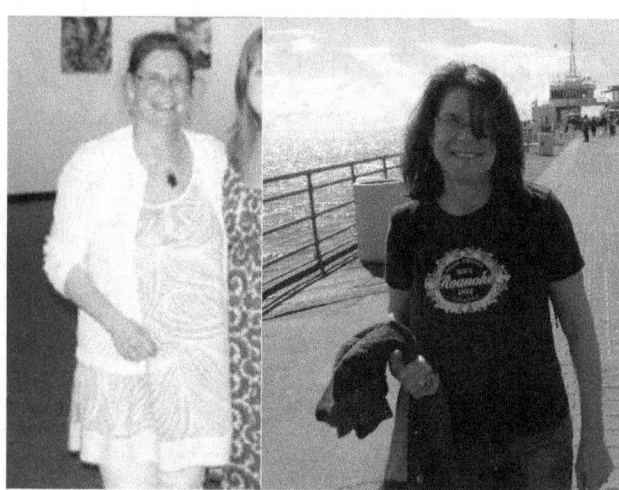

"I lost over 40lbs with the color-coding secret--who would have thought I could keep eating quesadillas?!

Now I use this method about once a month just to keep me on track.

Life is good!"

Ronda Kohn
Salem, VA

My mother was going through a challenging time in life.

Amongst the stress divorce, diving into her career so that she could have her own house, and handling two kids – one of which was a complete handful (I was the good one ☺) – her weight and gotten outta hand. Over a handful of years, she put on 40 extra lbs.

One year as a present I gave her a gift certificate to do my weight loss program, and she ordered her first week of free food.

She was *BAFFLED* after her first week. She lost 6lbs in 7 days, didn't do any exercise that week, and <u>couldn't believe that she was able to do it eating things like brownies & pasta.</u>

She stuck to it, and **was able to quickly drop the 40lbs**.
The most amazing part of the story is that she learned the **<u>3 step golden Weight Loss Success Strategy</u>**, and has used it ever since!

She's lean, and most importantly, she smiles all the time now. ← My favorite success story!

===================================

Bonus Resource

Now that you've got a full understanding of How to Lose Weight, you are now equipped to get quick results starting right away!

And just in case you're a tad overwhelmed by all of the info you just consumed, I want to make sure you have all the resources available to help you get started and see the process through.

So I created this for you...

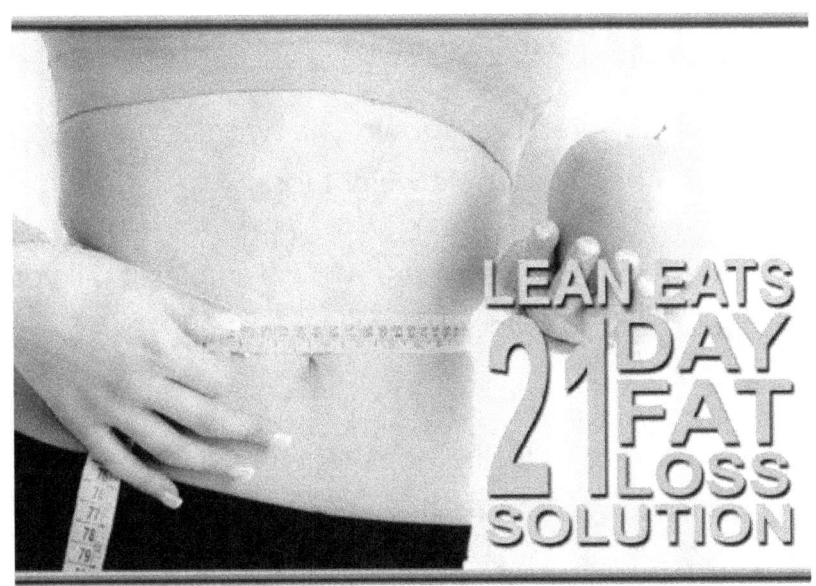

You'll want to take a look at this!

It's packed with tons of stuff that goes hand-in-hand with the info you've just learned.

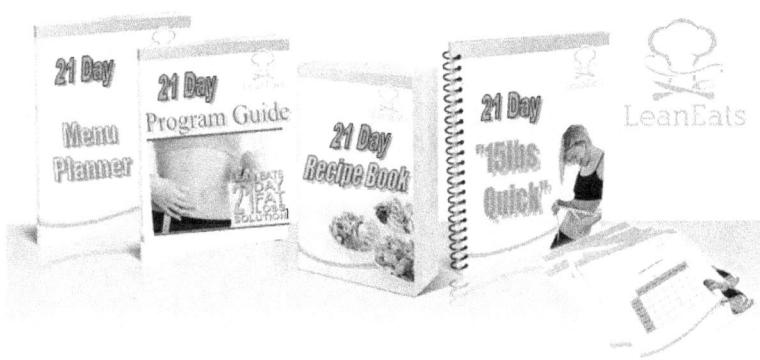

This program comes with:

- A Step-by-step breakdown of how to color code your meals for simple weight loss

- Menu Planner, with already DFY templates, all you have to do is follow the menu plan!

- **FULL 80 page Recipe book** (each meal is color coded so you can easily design a menu)

- **Mini-ebook on** the Science of Carb Cycling

- Program Schedule (walks you through step-by-step of what to do each day & week)

- *BONUS* you'll get a FREE Program Design phone call with the Lean Eats Nutrition Advisor, Roger Waddell! (He will answer all questions, and make sure you know *EXACTLY* what to do each day to get the best results.)

- *BONUS #2* *AND*, as a gift for checking out my book, for a very limited time, you can get it for **50% off**!!

If this sounds like what you need to get started so that you don't have to think – just start eating and get results now, I recommend picking this up before it goes off sale.

I don't want you to miss out on this opportunity (50% off!!)
because the sale is ending soon, and it goes back to normal price!

Check it out Here

www.myleaneats.com/#!21-day-fat-loss-solution/c1lvc

www.ingramcontent.com/pod-product-compliance
Lightning Source LLC
Chambersburg PA
CBHW060630290526
45793CB00001B/208